CeliacLost

A Family Guide to Finding a
——— Gluten-Free Life ———

Thanks Cheri!

Shelly &
Christopher

CeliacLost

A Family Guide to Finding a
Gluten-Free Life

Shelly Shiflett and Christopher Shiflett

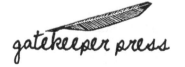

gatekeeper press

Columbus, Ohio

Celiac Lost: A Family Guide to Finding a Gluten-Free Life

Published by Gatekeeper Press
2167 Stringtown Rd, Suite 109
Columbus, OH 43123-2989
www.GatekeeperPress.com

ISBN (paperback): 9781642377002
eISBN: 9781642376999

Library of Congress Number: Pending

Celiac Lost website: www.celiaclost.com

We dedicate this book to our family and friends who have supported us on this journey, and to the many families who are beginning their own gluten-free life.

About This Book

When our son, Christopher, was diagnosed with celiac disease in August 2015, we felt lost and confused. How could this be? The child ate bread, pasta, and cake. He had no symptoms! Except ... his growth rate had slowed. And he had this strange little rash. As a mom and pediatric nurse, I should have caught this sooner, right?

The signs and symptoms of celiac disease are varied and often unclear, with some symptoms noticeable and others only rearing their heads later. Receiving the diagnosis as a child or an adult can feel overwhelming and sad for some, and for others it is a significant relief to finally know the source of their distressing symptoms. In either case, turning to the world of gluten-free living requires much education as you have real and permanent restrictions to a food protein that is seemingly everywhere.

Whether you are beginning gluten-free living from a place of complete surprise or a welcome change, we are all in this together to learn how best to start a new lifestyle and weed through the new world of labels and cooking methods. Our family approached this book from a starting point where we felt lost and overwhelmed, moving toward the place we're now in, feeling educated and content. We wrote this book with two goals in mind:

- The first goal is to address how to switch to a gluten-free diet in a simple and straightforward manner, encouraging you to keep your family recipes using gluten-free ingredient substitutions. We provide quick tips on grocery shopping, cooking, and meal ideas that took us years to discover.

- Our second goal is to address the family and social complications that can arise when you have a restrictive diet with celiac disease. The diagnosis affects the entire family and, sometimes, friendships. We share our mistakes and successes in hopes it will make your transition smoother.

This is the book we wish we had when Christopher was diagnosed.

"Triage" Table of Contents

In nursing, 'triage' involves prioritizing patient treatment by degree of urgency. When you are diagnosed with celiac disease, your first urgent need is to find out what you can eat! After that key concern is addressed, you are ready to learn and take control of this new lifestyle. For the purposes of this book, we've tried to triage what celiac patients often want to know first, followed by what they can address later. *However, read this book in whatever order fits your needs or interests.*

Introduction: Our Story 11

Triage #1: EAT

Chapter 1: What to Eat NOW 19

Triage #2: LEARN

Chapter 2: Celiac Disease – The Basics and The Lists 23
Chapter 3: The Grocery Store and Labeling 31
Chapter 4: Prepare Your Home for the Gluten-Free
            and the Gluten-Loving 41
Chapter 5: Socializing the Gluten-Free Way............................ 49

Triage #3: TAKE CONTROL

Chapter 6: Your Recipe Approach: "Change ONE Thing" 57
Chapter 7: Everyday Gluten-Free Meal and Snack Ideas 69
Chapter 8: Christopher's Favorite Recipes 81

Helpful Resources.. 99
Acknowledgments 101
Bibliography.. 103

Our Story

The idea for this book came to me as I was taking a walk and thinking how Christopher has grown and taken ownership of his diagnosis. He has taught me so many things about gluten-free cooking. During the first two years of his diagnosis, Christopher would occasionally come to me with cooking ideas, tips, and recipes that were, time and time again, immensely helpful. He started to ask a lot of questions about how I was cooking things (what flour I was using, why this brand seemed to work better than that other brand, etc.), and little did I know that he had been viewing a lot of food channels and cooking websites. Christopher has advanced from "I don't like this" (fill in the blank . . . bread, pasta, etc.), or just not eating what I gave him, to "I'm going to fix biscuits this morning. I'm going to make spaghetti carbonara tonight." He has totally taken charge and done so through extensive research on his own. Christopher agreed we should share our experience and together we have collaborated on this book

As I reflect back on this entire experience, I've come to realize that we really have three stories to share: one as a parent of a child with celiac disease, one as the child experiencing the diagnosis, and another as a family. We all have different perspectives on this process, and I think sharing our individual stories can help others. This book is designed not only for people who have a new celiac disease diagnosis, but also for anyone who has a friend, family member, or loved one with the disease and wants to understand better and provide support.

Mom's Story:

I am the proud mother of two sons, Tyler and Christopher, who are currently teenagers. Like many moms and parents, I have found that having children fundamentally changed me as a person. The challenges and situations you find yourself in as a parent really make you focus on priorities and the importance of family. Being a parent also enhances the realization of how out of control we really are and how the decisions we make are an effort to regain a sense of control. I highlight this last point because, since having children, I have always tried to make something good happen out of whatever cards we are dealt—it is how I try to regain control of my world and figure out God's plan for us.

My children were both born prematurely. Tyler was seven weeks early, but Christopher was 12 weeks early despite my best efforts to stay pregnant full-term. Fortunately, his two months in the NICU went fairly smoothly other than the apnea (stop breathing) and bradycardia (slow heart rate) that occurred with his bottle feedings. While scary for me that we might have to resuscitate him during his meals, it was an expected condition of his prematurity and he grew out of it. Nonetheless it struck me that something so nurturing as feeding my child could be a life or death situation. This experience led me to change my career from business to nursing when he was one year old, and since then I have tried to positively apply both my knowledge and attitude to 'out of control situations' to ones of growth and opportunity. So I find it interesting today, with Christopher's diagnosis of celiac disease (once again, feeding my child can cause danger and damage), that I continue to work to gain control and find resilience in the challenges we are presented.

For our family, the diagnosis was a surprise and yet another "out of control" moment. We had no family members with the disease and were generally unfamiliar with it. Christopher never complained of gastrointestinal symptoms, and he had no overt signs other than delayed growth. So our initial reaction to the news was one of sadness and, to a certain extent, we went through a grieving process. The sadness came from realizing that Christopher will have to live his life differently from most people when it comes to food. He will have to look at food suspiciously now, ask a lot of questions, and protect himself, all at an age and time when he just wants to fit in and not be different.

Additionally, we believed we had to say goodbye to a multitude of favorites and family recipes—bread, pasta, cake, cookies, sandwiches, crackers, etc. I remember standing at the entrance of the grocery store one day and realizing almost every item I saw had gluten in it. *He can eat nothing in here,* I thought. That was just overwhelming to me, and I felt utterly lost as a parent.

Immediately after he was diagnosed, I started to piece together all the signs I'd missed over the previous 13 years of Christopher's life (otherwise known as the 'mom guilt phase'). Christopher never complained of stomach pain, but he spent extra time in the bathroom, particularly after visiting our favorite Mexican restaurant. He was never an 'allergic' kid, but all of a sudden he was breaking out in hives (turns out he was allergic to pine nuts linked to peanut butter) and had a mysterious rash that came and went on its own. A routine blood test at his annual physical once identified anemia, but it resolved with the addition of iron-fortified vitamins. For Christopher, the primary sign of a possible health problem was the decline in his growth pattern from the third percentile to below the first. This drop in height velocity prompted another blood test which revealed indicators for celiac. The endoscopic biopsy confirmed the diagnosis, and our journey began.

After the guilt phase, I found myself going into overdrive to 'solve the problem.' I immediately went online to order a gluten-free recipe book. However, after reviewing the recipes I realized that in addition to this major change of no gluten (that seemed to be in everything we ate), I would now be introducing brand-new recipes to our family, with ingredients we had never used in the past. I held off buying the cookbook, hoping I could find a way to keep our current recipes. My second move was to buy anything and everything labeled 'gluten-free.' I had no idea how to shop the grocery store correctly and for me it was just easier to get things blatantly labeled gluten-free than to read, research, and compare all the food. All this new information was too much—too many rules, too much hidden gluten, too many things I didn't know yet. So, purely out of fear, and to keep things simple, I eventually just forced the entire family to eat everything gluten-free. My overdrive approach left other members of the family feeling alienated and ignored.

Whatever you and your loved ones are feeling regarding this diagnosis, know this: it is entirely normal. Whether you are happy to have a diagnosis finally or are dreading the change to a completely gluten-free life, you should know that you can make these changes successfully. It just takes some extra education, thought, and planning. I believe the most effective approach to making this change is to try to keep your traditions and family recipes as much as possible. You will find that often you can keep meals almost the same if you just change one thing—one ingredient or one method of preparation.

In this book, we have shared stories of our experience, mistakes, and successes in the hope that you can make your transition easy and quick. It's natural to feel overwhelmed (and scared) by all the information available through the internet, books, and friends. If you can find sources that make your life easier and simpler, you'll feel happier and more in control. You can do this!

Christopher's Story:

When I was first told that I had celiac disease, I didn't know what it was. My mother explained it to me while we were sitting in the kitchen and I asked if I could have cheese and crackers. She said no, so I asked if I could have ramen noodles or ravioli. She said no to both, and it felt like my life was falling apart. It seemed like I couldn't eat anything. I began learning the specifics of celiac disease by looking up the diagnosis online and talking with my mom. Over the first year I learned how to live a normal life while coming to understand the challenges I could encounter from eating certain ingredients.

When I told my friends about my diagnosis, they all wanted to know what it was. Fortunately for me, they seemed indifferent about it and we have moved on, other than the occasional joke about food here and there. Many of the people I tell about celiac assume you can't have regular food items such as bread or pasta, so I have to tell them about other flours like corn, rice, tapioca, etc. and how you can adapt. That's why we've created this book.

I want to help others by writing about our experience and educating people about celiac disease. My advice to others first diagnosed with celiac disease is that there are a lot of gluten-free alternatives. You will feel better about the food and diagnosis over time. Researchers are continuing to work on a cure and options that will make our lives easier. Until the research catches up, I hope you'll join my mom and me to learn about how you can feel in control and still enjoy food.

Our Family Story:

When we received the phone call with Christopher's diagnosis, I immediately called my husband to discuss. Not having much initial knowledge on celiac disease, we quickly decided we would just change our household diet and move forward. What we never considered, however, is the impact the diet change and restrictions would have on our son, Tyler, who does not have a problem with gluten. We confess it never occurred to us to have a proper meeting or 'training' with our family as a whole—to discuss the diagnosis, talk about concerns, or plan how we would approach this going forward. Over time, our family paid an unfortunate price with some hurt feelings and miscommunication.

I remember breaking the news to Christopher one afternoon while we were sitting in the kitchen. He was very disappointed—but he was ready to move on, trust me, and help figure it out. What I forgot to do, however, is adequately inform and educate Tyler. I'm not sure I explained anything to him. I think I just forced everything upon him as a "do this," "do that," and gave him a look if he hesitated to eat anything gluten-free. I remember Tyler one day saying to me, months after Christopher's diagnosis, that he had "nothing to eat . . . it's all gluten-free." This sent me over the edge, of course, so I went to the pantry, irritated. I realized that every time I went to the grocery store, I bought everything that said "gluten-free." The gluten-free section of our pantry was literally overflowing, and mostly uneaten. Tyler's gluten section had significantly diminished . . . I was almost completely ignoring him and his favorites. Still, I discounted his complaints since he could eat anything and should be thankful!

Finally, Tyler voiced his feelings again that everything was focused on Christopher, and he no longer had a say in his own food. I broke down and, in tears, said, "I'm doing the best that I can!" I realize now that I never took the time to have a real discussion with Tyler, never answering his questions, concerns, and the impact this change in his brother's diet would have on him. I honestly did an awful job with this transition, which is why we strongly encourage families to find ways to educate, support, and really listen to each other. The benefit of discussing the diet—either one-on-one or as a family or both—is that the transition will be more successful, and gluten-loving people will be much more aware and knowledgeable with their family and with their friends who may also have celiac disease. Overall we have each learned it is essential to listen to and treat the gluten-free and gluten-loving equally, and try to make reasonable accommodations as best as possible. As a family we should all be able to coexist and eat at the table together; it just requires patience and empathy.

CHAPTER 1 ⸻

What to Eat NOW?

When first diagnosed with celiac disease, understanding what you can eat – and cannot – is important. We are not used to thoroughly reading every label, understanding how food is processed, and automatically knowing the key words of "gluten" which are primarily wheat, rye, barley and malt (although there are many more key words listed in Chapter 2).

To help make this process easier, we have created a quick and easy chart to get you started (see next page). When using this chart, please remember these basic rules:

1. Start eating fresh, whole foods (minimally processed) – fruits, vegetables, meats, dairy, grains and legumes (like plain rice, beans, etc) are naturally gluten-free.
2. If a food has a label, read it. Stay away from wheat, barley, rye and malt. Maltodextrin is not malt and is gluten-free.
3. The safest gluten-free food has a Certified Gluten-Free label or says 'gluten-free' on package. But not all gluten-free food is required to have this certification (see Chapter 3).

In your home currently, it is important to know what is NOT safe to eat:

1. Your regular bread, cookies, crackers, pasta, etc. Read the label to get used to identifying gluten.
2. Any food or condiment in a jar/container that is used multiple times has gluten crumbs in it and therefore is cross-contaminated (ie, butter, jam, peanut butter, mayonnaise, etc.). Buy fresh jars and use squeeze bottles.
3. Check your combination spices – taco, pot roast, bouillon cubes, chili seasoning, etc. – for wheat or malt. Change manufacturers for gluten-free spices.
4. Canned soups often contain gluten. Read labels.

The following chart lists all the foods you can eat NOW!

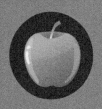

ALL FRESH FRUITS
(Oranges-Apples-Bananas-ETC)

Jams and jellies are usually gluten-free. Your current jams are likely cross-contaminated with gluten bread crumbs after multiple uses. Start with fresh jams.

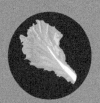

ALL FRESH VEGETABLES
(Lettuce-Cucumbers-Carrots-ETC)

Package salads with croutons or tortilla strips can contaminate the salad. Make sure to double check salad dressings for gluten.

ALL FRESH MEATS
(Beef-Chicken-Pork-Seafood-ETC)

Marinated meat can have gluten - make sure to read the label. Bacon, sausage, and deli meats often gluten-free. Verify with deli.

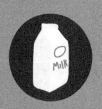

MOST FRESH DAIRY PRODUCTS
(Eggs-Milk-Cheeses-ETC)

Yogurts and ice cream can use wheat as a thickener or flavor additive. Malted chocolate is NOT gluten-free. Choose other chocolate milk options.

Can Eat NOW!

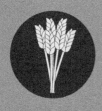

GRAINS AND LEGUMES
(Rice-Corn-Peanuts-Beans-ETC)

Flavored products can have wheat added. Oats can be exposed to gluten through processing, so look for gluten-free label.

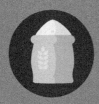

GLUTEN-FREE FLOUR, BREADS AND PASTA

Must say "gluten-free" on the label. Gluten-free all-purpose flour available, as well as single ingredient flour.

BEVERAGES
(Soda-Coffee-Tea-Fruit Juice-ETC)

Distilled liquors are often gluten-free. Most beers are not, unless labeled.

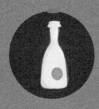

CONDIMENTS
(Ketchup-Oil-Butter-Spices-ETC)

Generally gluten-free. Current multi-use jars (peanut butter, mayo, butter) where multiple knives carrying crumbs are used can contaminate. Start with fresh jars.

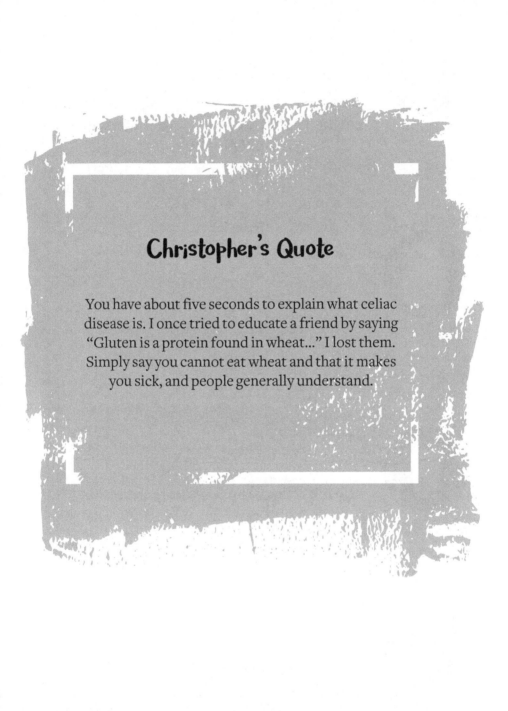

Christopher's Quote

You have about five seconds to explain what celiac disease is. I once tried to educate a friend by saying "Gluten is a protein found in wheat..." I lost them. Simply say you cannot eat wheat and that it makes you sick, and people generally understand.

CHAPTER 2 _____

Celiac Disease – The Basics and The Lists

Though our goal in writing this book isn't to dwell on the many medical details and pathophysiology of celiac disease—rather, we want to focus on the positive changes you can make—being a registered nurse, I know that the most effective transition to a new lifestyle requires a holistic approach. In our journey, I wanted to understand the basics as to what was going on in my child's body when he ate gluten, and I needed Christopher to understand as well. The damage occurring to his body was significant and he was not gaining nutritional value from his meals. In this section, we'll briefly review the known facts regarding celiac disease and foods containing gluten. As always, refer to your own gastroenterologist and dieticians for more detail and medical updates.

Celiac disease is an autoimmune disorder that is triggered by the ingestion of gluten commonly found in wheat, rye, and barley. When a person with celiac disease ingests gluten, the immune system attacks the small intestine, which in turn damages the villi, the small fingerlike projections along the intestine lining. Damage to the villi means a person is unable to absorb nutrients from food and can lead to a cascade of medical conditions.

Symptoms of celiac disease vary greatly from person to person and therefore the condition is underdiagnosed. Many times the diagnosis comes in adulthood. Symptoms can include gastrointestinal signs such as abdominal distention, diarrhea, and vomiting, as well as non-gastrointestinal signs like iron-deficiency anemia, osteoporosis, a herpetic rash, dental enamel defects, delayed growth and puberty, depression, and fatigue. The current gold standard for diagnosis is a biopsy of the small intestine. Certain blood tests can screen for celiac disease, including genetic testing, but they are not diagnostic. Newer serology and blood tests are being developed, and those tests, along with evaluation of symptoms, may lead to a diagnosis without the invasive endoscopy. There are many online resources to learn more detail about celiac disease, but one of the best resources is the Celiac Disease Foundation, www.celiac.org, which has consolidated a lot of resources, including internet blogs and scientific research.

It is important to note that celiac disease is hereditary and can run in families. If a first-degree family member (parent, sibling, child) has a confirmed diagnosis, you may consider talking to your physician about having your family members take a screening test for celiac disease.

This disease is exclusively treated and controlled through diet—no pills, no shots. That said, being on a gluten-free diet can be cumbersome and expensive. Research has found that gluten-free diets can increase the cost of food by approximately one-third of normal. For example, gluten-free bread, baked goods, and flour can be two to five times the price of wheat-based items. Christopher's favorite sandwich bread is Udi's Gluten-Free Delicious Soft White bread. We pay anywhere from $8 to $12 per loaf. Compared to the average cost of regular bread, which is about $2.50, this is a 350 percent increase of a basic food item. Gluten-free flour mixes (three-pound bags) can be anywhere from $8 to $25 compared to regular wheat flour at $3.50 for a five-pound bag. When I realized this cost difference on essential food items, I was stunned at the impact on our budget. As a result, I now find myself being judicious and less wasteful when making gluten-free meals. Fortunately, the prices of gluten-free items continue to come down over time and more and more products and manufacturers are appearing.

As a final note regarding celiac disease and the gluten-free diet, some people have found they continue to have symptoms or don't get enough relief from the new diet. If this is the case, you need to follow up with your physician and dietician to determine if any further allergy testing or blood work needs to be done, or a more thorough review of your diet. Annual health checkups with your gastroenterologist and dietician are crucial to staying healthy.

In order to eat gluten-free, you must not consume any food that contains wheat, barley, rye, or malt. Foods that are processed and labeled "gluten-free" must contain less than 20 ppm (20 parts of gluten per one million parts of food sample) of trace gluten in order to be considered safe for celiac patients.

Tale of Two Lists:

When we received the doctor's phone call confirming that Christopher had celiac disease, we immediately set up a dietician appointment. We fully expected our dietetic visit to be a lengthy meeting reviewing the many ways Christopher could easily adapt to a gluten-free diet and maybe we would learn some new recipes. In fact, I had already changed his diet and recorded all the gluten-free meals I fixed for him, and proudly presented my hard work and research to the dietician. To our dismay, the meeting was brief and consisted of the dietician handing us one sheet of paper containing two food lists, a series of concerns that I might still have exposed him to "hidden gluten," and general instructions to do research on the internet. I left concerned and frustrated because I expected the dietician to be more supportive and empathetic, and to provide more complete information instead of a single sheet with food lists and a blanket referral to the internet, which can often be scary and inaccurate. The meeting left me feeling uneasy and with little confidence that I could effectively navigate the world of gluten-free. As for Christopher, he says he barely remembers the meeting (he was age 13 at the time). He just wanted to trust me for direction on his meals and eating, but he soon began to research and figure out his diet on his own.

The lists the dietician gives you are relatively universal and are shown on the next two pages. This "list" moment is probably the most depressing part of your office visit. As discussed earlier, you feel a bit like you aren't allowed to eat anything and become concerned about all the hidden gluten in products. But be assured, after reading this book and understanding the food lists, food labels, and all the many substitutions available, you will find happiness in your gluten-free life.

List #1: Gluten-Containing Grains – THE HARD AND FAST LIST

AVOID at all times.

Barley

Bran

Bulgur

Couscous (a wheat)

Durum (a wheat)

Einkorn (a wheat)

Emmer (a wheat)

Brewer's yeast

Seitan (wheat gluten)

Spelt (hulled wheat)

Udon (Japanese wheat pasta)

Rye

Farina (a milled wheat)

Faro (a wheat)

Graham flour

Kamut (a wheat)

Matzo flour or meal

Orzo (a pasta)

Panko*

Malt, malt extract, malt syrup

Semolina (a wheat)

Triticale (wheat & rye hybrid)

Wheat, wheat bran, wheat germ, wheat starch

Gluten-Free panko is available in grocery stores.

List #2: Potentially Hidden Sources of Gluten (a.k.a. "everything else")

Bread/breading

Communion wafers

Lunchmeat

Roux

Stuffing

Soy sauce

Beer and lagers

Play-Doh

Adhesives

Coating mix

Lipstick, gloss, and balms

Brown rice syrup

Croutons

Broth

Sauces

Self-basting poultry

Marinades

Vitamin and mineral supplements

Toothpaste

Candy

Pasta

Soup base

Medications: Prescription and Over-the-Counter

Imitation seafood

Meat substitutes (imitation bacon, veggie burgers, etc.)

What Christopher and I have learned over the past four years is that the first list is "hard and fast", meaning you can't eat wheat, barley, rye, or variations which have gluten. However, the second list with potentially hidden sources of gluten (like soy sauce, candy, and toothpaste) has many alternatives and substitutions. For example, you can easily have soy sauce if you choose a different manufacturer. The second list propelled us to write this book because we initially took it at face value and it felt like there were no foods left to eat. The truth is there are many gluten-free options within List #2. Do you need to be aware of potentially gluten-containing products? Yes. Are there alternatives to each item on this list? Yes. That's what we're here for, and our goal is to make your life easier.

LIST YOUR HEALTH PROVIDERS AND RESOURCES

_____

_____

_____

_____

_____

_____

_____

_____

_____

_____

_____

_____

_____

_____

_____

_____

_____

_____

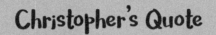

Christopher's Quote

My opinion: Gluten-free bread is demoralizing. When you first change your diet, don't introduce a lot of gluten-free processed food (like bread, donuts, etc.). Instead start with natural gluten-free foods like meat, vegetables, fruits, rice, corn, and potatoes. Gradually try the gluten-free breads and processed foods. Eventually you will get used to the taste and texture.

CHAPTER 3 ──────────────────

The Grocery Store and Labeling

One of the first things we did when we learned of the celiac diagnosis was go to the grocery store. We chose to go to an organic grocery store because what other place screams "gluten-free"? Having zero knowledge of how to find and evaluate gluten-free foods, we strolled through the aisles expecting gluten-free labels to jump out at us. But everything, it seemed, had gluten in it: the 'fresh' prepared meals. Yogurt. Prepared salads. Shredded cheese. When we eventually found the gluten-free section, the area was tiny. Itty bitty. This was concerning. We didn't know how we were going to choose foods we enjoyed eating with such a limited selection. We left the store confused, and with just a few groceries.

This experience taught us how little we knew about food and food labeling. If it wasn't labeled "gluten-free," *was* it gluten-free? Could we trust the labeling? Did people at the grocery store actually know what we were talking about when asked, "Is it gluten-free?" Because most of them looked thoroughly confused when asked the question, or they acted like they knew when they clearly did not.

Thus, we thought we should summarize our grocery store experiences so that you don't have to go through what we did. The aimless wandering down the aisles ends here! Learn the general rules with food labeling and move on.

> Hint #1: Gluten-free food is available throughout the entire grocery store, not just in one section. Many more options are available online.

Hint #2: Your key words for identifying gluten in food are: wheat, rye, barley, malt, or malt extract. (Note: maltodextrin is safe.)

Hint #3: Gluten-free food is not always labeled "gluten-free."

The Law and Labeling

The U.S. Food and Drug Administration (FDA) requires, by law, that all food manufacturers identify eight food allergens in the ingredients' section of packaging: wheat, milk, eggs, fish, crustacean shellfish, peanuts, tree nuts, and soybeans. Interestingly the FDA says that there are at least 160 foods that can cause allergic reactions, but 90 percent of the reactions are caused by the eight allergens listed above. Most of the food you buy is regulated by the FDA and will have a label with allergens listed.

The United States Department of Agriculture (USDA) monitors certain other foods such as poultry, most meats, and certain egg products (like dried, frozen, or liquid eggs). These products are currently not required to have allergen labeling (although they often include allergen labeling). Additionally, alcohol (including wine and beer) is controlled by the Bureau of Alcohol, Tobacco, and Firearms (ATF) and is currently not required to be labeled with allergens. However, alcoholic beverages are starting to follow FDA guidelines to give consumers more information.

Because there are several agencies regulating our food, it is important to educate yourself on what food is and is not required to be labeled and what the basic gluten-containing foods are so you know what foods are safe. As a reminder, in order for a product to be considered gluten-free it must contain less than 20 parts per million of gluten.

If you would like more detail on food allergy label requirements, visit the FDA website at www.fda.gov, the USDA website at www.usda.gov, and the ATF at www.atf.gov. Other great resources on food labeling and information on celiac disease include the Celiac Disease Foundation at www.celiac.org and Beyond Celiac at www.beyondceliac.org.

How to Identify Gluten-Free Foods

The required FDA labeling is immensely helpful to those with allergies, but it doesn't eliminate additional reading and knowledge on your part.

In order to identify a food as gluten-free, follow these methods:

Method 1 – No Label:
You already know the food is naturally
gluten-free even though it has no label.

Method 2 – Labeled Gluten-Free:
The food is clearly labeled "gluten-free" either
with words or symbols on its package.

Method 3 – Read the Label:
The food label identifies key words to indicate the
presence or absence of gluten ingredients: wheat,
rye, barley, or malt. (See also Chapter 2 lists).

Details of the Methods

Method 1 – No Label:
These are foods in their natural, whole state: fruits, vegetables, meats, eggs, milk, etc. These items will not have a label, but you know they are naturally gluten-free. If these items are further processed and have a label, read it.

Method 2 – Labeled Gluten-Free:
Foods are processed and clearly identified as gluten-free (like gluten-free pasta and bread). Food manufacturers have a variety of ways to inform customers about gluten-free; there isn't one uniform way.

a) Look for the words "gluten-free" written either in the title of the item or somewhere on the packaging. "Gluten-free fettuccine" is an example.

b) Look for a gluten-free symbol on the package. Symbols or pictures are created either by a certifying agency or the manufacturer and are not uniform. Certifying agencies include the Gluten-Free Certification Organization and NSF International. If a gluten-free symbol is created by the food manufacturer (versus the certifying agencies mentioned), it means you're trusting the manufacturer to ensure products are truly gluten-free. In general, we trust such labels because the manufacturers are still under the auspices of the FDA and allergy-labeling requirements. If you have questions or want to thoroughly research products, you can go to the manufacturer's website or to celiac or gluten-free dedicated websites. There are also some independent organizations such as Gluten-free Watchdog who voluntarily test various gluten-free products in the marketplace to ensure they are truly gluten-free.

Method 3 – Read the Label:
If the food doesn't include the words or symbol for gluten-free, or you know it's not naturally gluten-free (because it's processed), then you need to read the ingredient list. Within the ingredient list, the manufacturer will state ingredients in one of the following ways:

Method 3 (continued):

    a)   Gluten is stated directly within the ingredient list (e.g., malt).
           NOT SAFE to eat

Ingredients: Rice, sugar, contains 2% or less of salt, malt flavor. ←

Vitamins and Minerals: Iron (ferric phosphate), vitamin C (ascorbic acid), vitamin E acetate, niacinamide, vitamin A palmitate, vitamin B_6 (pyridoxine hydrochloride), vitamin B (thiamin hydrochloride), vitamin B_2 (riboflavin), folic acid, vitamin B_{12}, vitamin D_3.

Ingredientes: Arroz, azúcar, contiene 2% o menos de sal, sabor malta.

    b)   The food packaging lists each ingredient and at the end states, often in bold type, "Allergens: wheat, etc." **NOT SAFE to eat**

Ingredients: Corn, Whole Grain Wheat, Sugar, Whole Grain Rolled Oats, Rice, Dried Apples, Canola Oil, Wheat Flour, Malted Barley Flour, Cinnamon, Corn Syrup, Salt, Molasses, Honey, Barley Malt Extract, Natural Flavor. BHT added to preserve freshness.

Vitamins and Minerals: Reduced Iron, Niacinamide (Vitamin B3), Zinc Oxide, Thiamin Mononitrate (Vitamin B1), Pyridoxine Hydrochloride (Vitamin B6), Folic Acid.

CONTAINS WHEAT. ←

c) The food packaging lists each ingredient, none of which may be gluten-containing, but at the end, the package states "has been processed in a facility that has wheat, nuts, etc." Thus, the product is considered contaminated and not gluten-free.

INGREDIENTS: RAISINS, ROASTED, NO SALT SUNFLOWER SEEDS (VEGETABLE OIL [COTTONSEED OIL AND/OR SUNFLOWER OIL]), ROASTED, NO SALT ALMONDS (ALMONDS, CANOLA OIL), ROASTED NO SALT PUMPKIN SEEDS (PUMPKIN SEEDS, CANOLA OIL), ROASTED, NO SALT CASHEWS (CASHEWS, CANOLA OIL). CONTAINS TREE NUTS (ALMONDS, CASHEWS). PACKED IN A FACILITY THAT USES PEANUTS, TREE NUTS, MILK, SOY, EGGS AND WHEAT.

Keep in mind that the most up-to-date ingredient list is on the product at the store, but the internet is also helpful. As an additional resource, use your phone to research products, read up on the manufacturer, and the product's current gluten-free status. Just type in "Is _____ gluten-free?" for helpful information.

If the food product identifies its ingredients, there is no gluten in the ingredient list or under "allergens," and you're comfortable (through your research) that the ingredients don't contain gluten, then it should be safe to eat. There are always caveats, but if you stay educated and read labels, you'll be fine.

While initial trips to the grocery store may be longer due to research and reading, utilizing these methods will shorten them. Rest assured your grocery shopping will not always be so time-consuming. Your research and understanding now will save you time in the future!

"Organic," "Non-GMO," and "Vegan" do NOT mean Gluten-Free

We never thought of this labeling as confusing until we were at a dinner and one guest proudly announced that the pasta dish in front of us was "non-GMO" and we should help ourselves! Apparently the presence of the letter "G" within the special "labeling" was enough to assume it meant gluten-free. Alternatively, many people mistake processed foods labeled as "organic" as also being gluten-free. This is *not* the case.

Gluten-free foods can be organic, non-GMO, and vegan, but identifying a food item as organic, non-GMO, or vegan does not automatically mean it is also gluten-free. Always read the labels.

Shop the Perimeter ... Mostly

The old adage "shop the perimeter" of your grocery store as the way to get the healthiest foods is true, but keep in mind that the bakery, pizza shop, and processed refrigerated items are also located there! However, you can shop the perimeter for fresh fruits, vegetables, meats, and dairy which are naturally gluten-free.

Summary of gluten-free foods:

☞ Fresh fruits and vegetables.

☞ Fresh and minimally processed meats (beef, chicken, pork, seafood, etc.) that are not imitation or processed into something else (for example, meatballs) and are free from marinades and broths.

☞ Most deli meats. Talk to your deli to ensure gluten-free.

☞ Most dairy products (with no add-ins) including eggs, milk, cheese, sour cream, cottage cheese, ricotta cheese, and cream cheese. Yogurts can contain thickeners, so look for a gluten-free label. Ice creams tend not to have a gluten-free label/symbol, so read ingredient lists.

☞ Nuts, beans, and rice, unless combined with other ingredients that can contain gluten (like trail mix or flavored rice). This grouping sometimes has a label statement "processed in facility that has exposure to wheat, gluten, etc." and in such cases the product is not safe.

☞ Oils (olive, canola, etc.), butter, and vinegars. Spray oil with flour is not safe.

☞ Condiments (mustard, ketchup, mayonnaise, etc.). Avoid multi-use jars (containers where multiple utensils or foods containing gluten can cross-contaminate, making them unsafe).

☞ Fresh spices and dried individual spices. Check combination spices.

☞ Boxed broth is usually labeled gluten-free.

☞ Flours, breads, and pastas must say gluten-free. See Chapter 6 for details.

☞ Most drinks such as water, orange juice, limeade, sodas, fruit juices, club soda, sports drinks, etc. are safe.

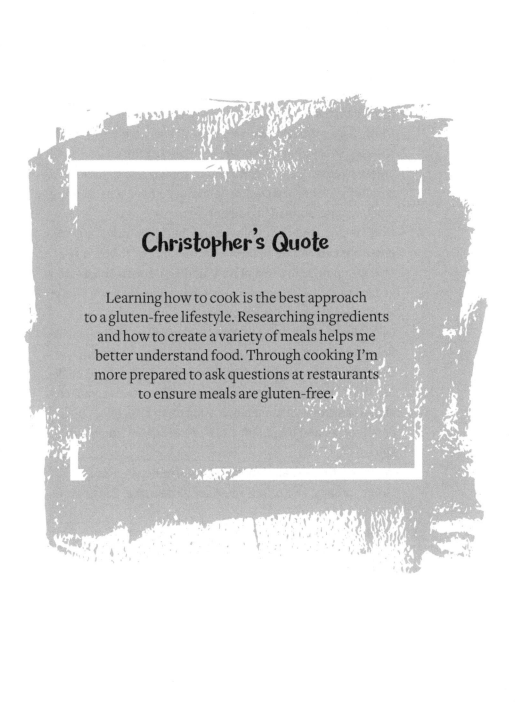

Christopher's Quote

Learning how to cook is the best approach
to a gluten-free lifestyle. Researching ingredients
and how to create a variety of meals helps me
better understand food. Through cooking I'm
more prepared to ask questions at restaurants
to ensure meals are gluten-free.

CHAPTER 4 _____

Prepare Your Home for the Gluten-Free _and_ the Gluten-Loving

Having one (or more) persons in your home with celiac disease means the entire family must be educated because cross-contamination of gluten-filled crumbs or flour dust with gluten-free food can mean an unhealthy reaction for your loved one. The good news is there are reliable ways you can prepare your home to prevent accidental exposure. Reviewing the following tips as a family will inform everyone and help avoid accidental gluten ingestion. Family involvement is key to making this dietary transition successful.

Our suggestions for creating a gluten-free environment at home:

> _If you're feeling overwhelmed by all this information, take a break and a deep breath. We, also, felt overwhelmed by too much information – it was as if we couldn't change fast enough for Christopher's health and I felt like I was making mistakes all over the place. Sometimes I had to take mental breaks from all the reading, researching, and preparing. If you are feeling this way, please know you do NOT have to do everything at once. Focus on the small things that can be changed first and learn a little bit each day. Your loved one didn't get celiac disease overnight and you can't learn to deal with it overnight. Give yourself a break. Pick your priority each day (or week) and know you'll get there._

1. **CLEAN:** Give your kitchen countertops, tables, and cabinet/refrigerator handles a thorough cleaning. When gluten-containing foods touch a surface, even if no crumbs are visible, it is contaminated. Consider having a designated gluten-free

countertop area. Keep all surfaces clean by using paper towels and disinfectant. Wash your hands (and countertops) in between preparing foods that have gluten. Remember, your hands, as well as utensils, can transfer gluten, so keep aware of what you're touching.

2.   **DEDICATED APPLIANCE:** There are only two items we recommend you add to your kitchen. If possible, consider having a dedicated gluten-free toaster or toaster oven. Your gluten-free family member will use this appliance a lot and it is very worthwhile. If you're unable to have a separate one, you'll need to thoroughly clean your toaster/toaster oven after every use to ensure it is free of any wheat or gluten crumbs (seen or unseen). The other item we suggest is a dedicated colander for gluten-free pasta. When I make pasta dishes, I cook both regular pasta and gluten-free pasta in separate pots. If I don't have a second colander, I need to make sure the gluten-free pasta is cooked and ready first so it can use the colander first; then I transfer that pasta back to the pot and get ready for the gluten pasta.

3.   **EVALUATE POTS, PANS, AND BAKEWARE:** We have not found that we need separate pots and pans for effective gluten-free eating. Just be sure to clean these items thoroughly and switch out your kitchen sponges frequently (in fact, switch to a new sponge now). There is a concern that if your pot, pan, or bakeware has scratches in it, the scratch area could possibly house gluten (if you use them for both types of cooking). In that case, you may want to dispose of the damaged cookware. If you have the money and space, you could choose to have separate cookware. However, it does not appear to be necessary.

4. **CHECK YOUR CURRENT SPICES AND SEASONINGS:** As mentioned previously, pay particular attention to your "combination spices" like taco seasoning, grilling seasoning, chili powder, and packet spices including instant gravies and pot-roast seasoning. I had to throw out almost all of my combination spices because they had gluten. The good news is you can easily replace them with similar gluten-free seasoning options or make your own seasonings.

5. **CHECK YOUR CURRENT BROTHS:** Bouillon cubes and pastes you have used in the past likely contain gluten or may have been cross-contaminated. Double-check them and throw out if necessary. You'll find clearly labeled gluten-free broth and bouillon at the grocery store or online. (We cover this item in more detail in Chapter 6.)

6. **ORGANIZE YOUR PANTRY:** Inventory your pantry for gluten. If you have gluten lovers in your household, we recommend that you don't throw out their favorite foods! Instead, consider reorganizing your pantry between gluten-containing items and gluten-free items so your loved ones easily see what foods are available to them and what is off-limits. Also, consider gluten-free foods that may have been cross-contaminated such as a half-eaten jar of peanut butter. Put them in the "gluten area" and purchase a brand-new peanut butter for the "gluten-free" area. Mark each jar (with a "G" for gluten, maybe) for clarity.

7. **REVIEW AND ORGANIZE YOUR REFRIGERATOR AND FREEZER:** In the same way you inventoried your pantry, do the same with your refrigerator. In particular, review all of your current condiments for possible cross-contam-

ination: ketchup, mustards, mayonnaise, sour creams, yogurts, pickles, salad dressings, marinades, jams and jellies, hummus tubs, family butter dishes, etc. Squeeze bottles have less of a chance of gluten contamination, but consider your family's habits. Do they use knives to scrape the squeeze bottle or tend to wipe the last bit of squeeze bottle mayo on the bread of their sandwich? If you're unsure or just want to start fresh, then move all possibly cross-contaminated items to your gluten section. As an example, my refrigerator has a dual butter area in the door. I use the one on the left as a dedicated butter dish and butter area for gluten-free cooking. I use the second butter area for the gluten side of the family and have a dedicated butter stick and butter tub. If I have condiments that may be cross-contaminated, I mark the container with a "G" and inform family members.

8. **OTHER POSSIBLE GLUTEN IN THE HOUSE:** Consider other areas of the house that may have gluten:

    a) Dog or cat food may contain gluten. Be sure to wash your hands immediately after handling pet food.
    b) Toothbrushes and toothpaste can contain gluten or be cross-contaminated. Do a quick search online for toothpaste that is gluten-free (most are). To be safe, discard your current toothbrushes and toothpaste and start fresh.
    c) Medications and vitamins can contain gluten. If there are medications that are taken on a consistent or periodic basis (either over the counter or prescription) check the ingredient list and talk to your local pharmacist.

9. **FAMILY MEETING AND EDUCATION:** Once your kitchen has been prepared, have a family meeting to educate

and problem-solve. We strongly encourage you to be very thoughtful of each family member and think about the best way to communicate these important changes to your family's eating lifestyle. The person who must now eat gluten-free does not necessarily want to follow such a strict diet. More importantly, they don't want to feel different or blamed for changes. In the same vein, family members who don't require dietary restrictions will need to make changes to their daily habits, particularly when it comes to cross-contamination. They will now have to pay special attention when preparing and eating their food. Change can be difficult! So it's important that all family members are equally educated on celiac disease and see themselves as helpful partners.

We encourage you to make this dietary transition both educational and as positive as possible. Perhaps the family meeting should be one-on-one and more individualized. Or maybe the family member with celiac disease wants to describe the family plan and educate everyone on gluten and the new pantry arrangement. Tailor your discussions to what will work best for your family. The gluten-free and gluten-loving can coexist peacefully, but mutual respect and education are required.

Here is another tip from our experience as a family: On occasion, consider some family meals that include a regular, gluten-filled option. Yes, this takes more work on the part of the preparer, but if I've learned anything from this experience it's that ignoring the basic needs or preferences of the child or family member who does not need any dietary accommodation leads to a lot of resentment and a lot less eating. So for example, on spaghetti night I make one sauce for everyone, but I make two different pastas—one regular spaghetti and one gluten-free. If we decide to have cheesy garlic bread on the side, I make two different ones using the two different breads. For our beef stroganoff dish (rec- ipe in Chapter 8), I make two homemade egg-noodle batches from scratch—one regular, one gluten-free. Is it more time and work? Yes. Is it worth it to have people feel special? Absolutely. I know as a mom this can be hard, and maybe right now with the initial diagnosis this isn't the time to tackle a complication of "two" of something. And I do not advocate doing this every meal, especially if most of the meal isn't much different than a regular gluten meal (for example a meal of London broil, baked potato, and steamed vegetables is already gluten-free). But I do recom- mend accommodating when you can, and recognizing there are various needs in the household. Eventually you will get to a place where you can handle it.

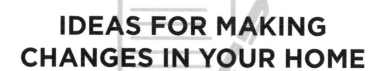

IDEAS FOR MAKING CHANGES IN YOUR HOME

_____

_____

_____

_____

_____

_____

_____

_____

_____

_____

_____

_____

_____

_____

_____

_____

_____

_____

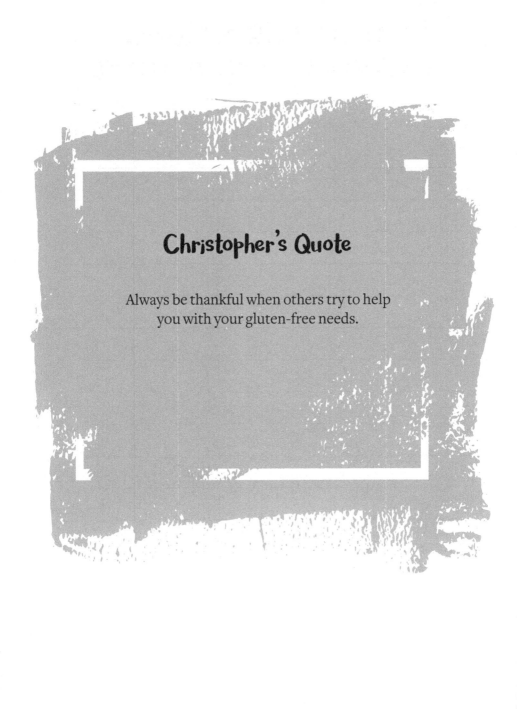

Christopher's Quote

Always be thankful when others try to help
you with your gluten-free needs.

CHAPTER 5 _____

Socializing the Gluten-Free Way

Besides the initial day-to-day family meal complications and adjustments you'll be making, you'll want to consider the impact being gluten-free may have on your social life. Eating is a social event, so the goal is to create a stress-free method of having social gatherings (at home or away) that accommodate your new lifestyle. You'll be warmly rewarded by opening up about being gluten-free with your friends and family.

Visiting Friends and Family Homes

One of the best experiences we have had is eating at a friend or family member's house. You may think that most people are not interested in celiac disease or do not want to take the time to find or fix gluten-free foods to accommodate this diet. For some people, this may be true. The majority of the time, though, your friends and family really want to help with your dietary transition and just need to know the basic rules. We have been absolutely blessed with Christopher's friends, their parents, and our family members who not only have accommodated his gluten-free living, but also clearly have done research on their own. They have come up with new recipes (or adjusted their own) and located gluten-friendly restaurants to ensure Christopher has a great experience and not feel so alone. We cannot thank them enough!!

Suggestions for socializing with friends and family:
1. Briefly explain to family or friends that you/your child/friend cannot have gluten, and that means no food with wheat (they may understand "flour" better), barley, rye, or malt.

2. Offer to pack food and bring a variety of gluten-free snacks, appetizers, entrees, etc. along when you visit. Make it as relaxed as possible. At a child/teen event, we supply snacks all kids tend to eat—potato chips, corn tortilla chips and salsa or queso, buffalo chicken dip, etc. If you bring rice cakes or some of the weird gluten-free crackers, it gets weird. Keep food as every day and "normal" as possible.

3. Often a host will want to try to make something on their own that is gluten-free and will just check with you on the ingredients. This is amazing! Depending on the meal, cross-contamination is possible. Don't panic. Thank them for their wonderful effort, inquire about their recipe, and if appropriate, as they're describing the dish, you can bring up cross-contamination. But we have found, in general, people do a great job with coming up with safe gluten-free recipes. And many times our friends and family have found new gluten-free options we didn't even know existed!

> *When your host wants to serve gluten-free:*
>
> *The first time this happened to us, I went into a panic. The host of our church's teen dinner called me to say she was going to cook gluten-free spaghetti. Aware of all the issues with cross-contamination, I quickly told her that I could supply Christopher's dinner. I then sensed the disappointment in her voice as she was clearly excited to try something new for him. I realized then that people want to help. Relax and let others in! Christopher enjoyed the meal, had no reactions, and introduced me to a new pasta I didn't know was available.*

4. Learn to say "no" to questionable foods, whether you are at a friend's house or a restaurant. If you feel unsure about other people's cooking, simply tell them, "thank you, but no". Explain that

you must be very cautious with your diet to prevent reactions. Your friends and family will understand, and they will be thankful that they will not be the cause of your gluten-induced symptoms.

5. Let your child/friend/family member with celiac disease take the lead in researching restaurants and recipes. It's important they continue to learn and give direct input on where they can eat, with ample options for their friends without dietary restrictions. Christopher is proactive with his friends in doing research on restaurants, and his friends are very accommodating and open. There have been a couple of instances where they have gone to a restaurant that claimed to be gluten-free and, after Christopher had a couple reactions, they willingly switched to a new restaurant.

One of the best outcomes we have experienced with Christopher's diagnosis is his desire to learn how to cook. One of the results of Christopher's creativity has been cooking contests with his friends. Yes, cooking contests! At first, I was disheartened when I learned that it was going to be a gluten-free dish versus a regular gluten-filled dish, a meal that he couldn't even taste to compare against his. A little unfair, I thought, given the caveats and creative adjustments you have to make with gluten-free cooking. But that was his point, he said. Christopher wanted to show others that a gluten-free meal can be just as good as a gluten-filled one. Brilliant! And risky. And bold. Awesome! Christopher knows that many of the gluten-free versions of bread and pasta simply don't match the original. But he's discovering flavorful and convenient alternatives on his own initiative, and creating amazing food.

Gatherings at Home

The obvious benefit of hosting parties at your home is that you're in control. After almost four years of working through the gluten-free lifestyle and hosting parties, I have learned that simple is best. I keep everything gluten-free because it's easier on me, and people won't know the difference. The main concern at parties is cross-contamination. Your guests don't need the complication of "don't dip THAT cracker into that dip. Use THIS cracker ..." So here are our suggestions for hosting parties:

- ☞ Convert your recipes to gluten-free or find new ones online. Chapter 6 provides detailed information on how to switch out gluten-free substitutions in your own recipes.
- ☞ When you cannot or do not want to use gluten-free substitutes, keep those items physically away from the gluten-free food. Let your loved ones know all the party foods they can eat. Prevent cross-contamination.
- ☞ Review Chapters 7 and 8 for meal ideas.

When we have Christopher's friends over, I generally keep everything gluten-free. This is easy because there are so many gluten-free snacks. For more substantial meals, I order regular pizzas for his friends and a separate gluten-free pie for Christopher. Call your local restaurants and ask about their gluten-free options and adherence to allergy protocol. If people want burgers and hot dogs, we can easily do that with the guests using regular buns and Christopher eating just the patty. It all works out very well. Be creative about all the food options available to you and keep these little events as simple as possible.

School Lunches

Talk directly to the teachers, administrators, and school cafeteria about your child's condition. In fact, the diagnosis of celiac disease can qualify your child for a 504 plan that requires accommodation. Websites such as the Gluten Intolerance Group and Beyond Celiac have resources and information to help you talk to schools about celiac disease, cross-contamination, and prevention. Teaching your child about their diagnosis and preventing contamination will go a long way to keeping them safe and knowledgeable. In terms of eating at school, our family has always chosen to bring their lunch, and from there we talk about preventing contamination (wash their hands before eating, keep their food away from others, only touch their own food, etc.). Please see Chapter 7 for meal ideas.

College Dining and Beyond

Just as important as deciding on a college, a major, dorm selection, and where you will feel most comfortable, you should also spend the same time learning about the gluten-free options at your university. Some colleges and college towns are better than others in terms of gluten-free friendliness. Be sure to take the time to research the dining facilities, access to kitchens in the dorms, refrigeration options (in room or kitchen), and popular local restaurants so you are clear on what your day-to-day life will look like and how it will accommodate healthy eating. Many universities have dining information online through dining services, and you can also talk to the school's dining director or manager. Research the local restaurants, review their menus, and email them about their gluten-free options and protocol. You want to feel confident and prepared that you can enjoy dining at college, both on and off campus. More helpful tips on college dining available online at the Food Allergy Research and Education website and the Beyond Celiac website.

Restaurants

Restaurants have increasingly improved each year with their knowledge, preparation, and gluten-free food options. The biggest danger with restaurants is cross-contamination by staff or cooks. Unfortunately you can't control this, but you can ask questions like "Are your french fries cooked in a separate fryer to keep gluten-free? Or do you cook all fried food in the same fryer?"

Research your restaurants online. Look at their menus and their disclaimers. You can also email them or call to get clarification.

The internet, restaurant guide books, and smartphone apps are great resources for finding restaurants with gluten-free options. One of the newest smartphone apps is called "Dedicated Gluten Free", and it focuses on helping you find 100% dedicated gluten-free eating establishments in your area or throughout the world. Another helpful app to download is "Find Me Gluten-Free". This application provides information on a variety of restaurants who offer gluten-free options (not always a dedicated facility) in your area. It is not an exhaustive list of every single restaurant that offers gluten-free, but it will give you many options. Keep updated on new smartphone applications by following Instagram, Facebook, and blog sites which are often the first to know. Just type in "celiac" or "gluten-free" in any of these portals and many helpful sites will come up.

NOTES

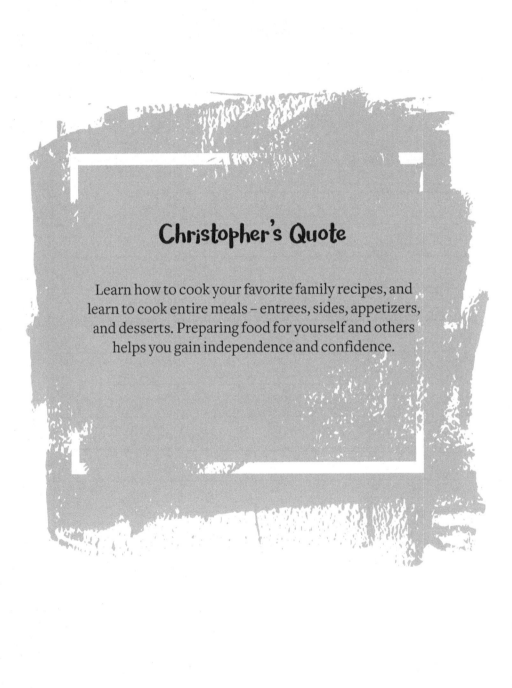

Christopher's Quote

Learn how to cook your favorite family recipes, and learn to cook entire meals – entrees, sides, appetizers, and desserts. Preparing food for yourself and others helps you gain independence and confidence.

CHAPTER 6 ———————————

Your Recipe Approach: "Change ONE Thing"

After researching and experimenting with gluten-free eating, we have identified two important insights that we want families—and maybe restaurants—to realize.

1. The vast majority of times, if you just change ONE ingredient or ONE method of food preparation/cooking, you have reopened a world of unfettered eating to a person with celiac disease. It's that simple. What makes the change to gluten-free cooking "difficult" is the fact that you have to read and think about food ingredients and preparation. However, once you make the necessary changes, gluten-free cooking becomes simple and easily adaptable.

2. *No food is truly off-limits (unless it's gluten).* Do you love pasta? Tons of gluten-free options. Bread? Yep, lots of celiac compliant choices. Cinnamon rolls are a favorite for you? We have a delicious homemade cinnamon roll recipe in Chapter 8. If you have celiac disease, do not take "no" for an answer. Be creative. You have a lot of options and substitutions available; it's just a matter of knowing what they are and adjusting to your personal preferences.

This section of the book is our collection of substitution ideas, tips, and recommendations on gluten-free food items and preparation. We want this to be a launching point for you to make quick, easy changes to your own family recipes.

As you read this chapter:

1. Look at your favorite recipes and identify ingredients that have gluten in them (for example flour, cream soup, spice pack, or pasta).
2. Find gluten-free replacements for those ingredients (check the options in this chapter).
3. Make your existing recipe using the gluten-free alternative.

Special Note: You can use any recipe (gluten-free, regular, or family). Don't feel limited to gluten-free recipes, although they often give insight into new ideas, new ingredients, and ways to prepare that you may not have thought of. As long as you know where gluten can exist and how to replace it, any recipe is available to you.

Gluten-free products are always improving and becoming more readily available. We encourage you to find great gluten-free substitutions through your local stores and online. Try a variety to see what you like best.

Basic Staples Used in Cooking and Baking

Flour:

> *Switch to gluten-free flour (either all-purpose or single ingredient) and continue with your current cooking and baking recipes.*

Flour is used in breads, cookies, pies, snacks, pasta, gravy, sauces, soups, and a multitude of processed products, so you'll want to know how best to substitute gluten-free flour into your life—quickly! What we didn't know about gluten-free flour is something you need to know right now:

1. All-purpose/multipurpose gluten-free flour exists as a replacement for regular wheat flour. Interestingly, gluten-free all-purpose flour is a combination of several different flours. You can use this flour, cup for cup, as a replacement for almost any recipe.

2. You can make your own all-purpose gluten-free flour by buying several individual flours and combining them. Instructions are available online.

3. Just about all gluten-free all-purpose flour combinations taste different and act different (unlike all-purpose wheat flours). Try several to see what you like.

4. Popular flours (like almond and coconut) are gluten-free, but generally not present in all-purpose flours. They are found in specific recipes.

5. Xanthan gum provides elasticity and stickiness to baked goods and needs to be in your all-purpose flour. Or at least you need to keep some on hand in a separate container.

There are several manufacturers of all-purpose flour, each with their own unique flour combinations, including cornstarch, white rice flour, brown rice flour, potato starch, and tapioca starch. Other flour mixes are made with garbanzo bean flour, pea fiber, and fava beans. As you can imagine, the taste and texture can vary between manufacturers of these all-purpose flours. It's important to know if your all-purpose flour contains xanthan gum or not. You'll need it in some recipes, and not all flour combinations include it. We like Cup4Cup for its taste,

When we received the diagnosis, we went to our local store and purchased individual bags of almond flour, brown rice flour, white rice flour, coconut flour, sorghum flour, tapioca starch, and xanthan gum at a combined cost of $48! Three years later, these flours are all still sitting in the pantry, virtually unused (except xanthan gum). When we realized there are all-purpose gluten-free flours, our world opened back up.

consistency, and lack of grittiness, but please try a variety of brands. Other manufacturers include but are not limited to King Arthur, Pillsbury, Bob's Red Mill, Arrowhead Mills, Better Batter, Firebird Artisan Mills, Hodgson Mill, and Pamela's products.

Special note about gluten-free flours:

☞ Wheat flours have a consistent taste. In contrast, gluten-free flours have a flavor reflective of the combination of flours used. For example, almond flour has a unique texture and nutty flavor in comparison to a flour made from cornstarch and rice.

☞ Texture and elasticity of baked products are different between wheat flour and gluten-free flours. Texture differences you may experience include grittiness (which is due to some flours like brown rice that are not as finely ground) and denser consistency.

☞ Using gluten-free flours often requires adjustments in the amount of liquid added, baking time, and cooling time (often so the baked good can "gel" better). Carefully follow the recommendations on the flour packaging or manufacturer suggestions for the best results.

The advances in gluten-free flours are always changing and improving. We recommend that you continue your research and experimentation with new flours and flour products available at your grocery store, online, or through gluten-free cookbooks.

🔎 Where to Find: Baking aisle and Gluten-free food aisle

Breads and Stuffing:

> *Switch to clearly labeled gluten-free bread, buns, bagel, and roll options and continue with your current sandwich and recipe favorites. Stuffing is also clearly labeled as gluten-free.*

After flour, bread is probably the most significant change when going gluten-free. We've tried dozens of bread options over the years, including baking our own and going to specialty bakeries. Gluten-free bread tastes different than regular wheat bread—often tasting like eggs or the majority flour ingredient. Its texture can be too light or too heavy, it's usually smaller in size, and it can fall apart very easily. There are books that tell you how to make the best gluten-free bread ever and provide all kinds of special instructions. Even so, if you love bread and bread-related products, transitioning to gluten-free bread is probably the biggest dietary adjustment you will make.

Examples of bread manufacturers:

Udi's, New Grains Gluten Free Bakery, Canyon Bakehouse (Canyon Gluten-Free), Franz, Glutino, Kinnikinnick, and Against the Grain. More gluten-free manufacturers are popping up all the time.

Quick Guide to Gluten-Free Bread:
- ☞ Give yourself time to find the brands and bread types you like best. For example, you may prefer one manufacturer for its sandwich bread, but like a different brand for making French toast. Gluten-free breads are always improving.
- ☞ Heating or toasting helps the taste and binding of most gluten-free breads. For school lunches, toast the bread (unless it's PB&J). Be sure to let the sandwich cool before packing it—otherwise, the condensation will break apart your beautiful gluten-free bread!
- ☞ After you purchase frozen bread, you can defrost and keep it in the refrigerator. You may consider putting it in a gallon bag to help retain its moisture. Read the label for recommended storage and preparation.

🔎 Where to Find: Frozen Bread aisle and Gluten-free frozen aisle

Broths:

Switch to gluten-free broth and continue using your current soup, marinade, and casserole recipes.

It's surprising how often broth is used in recipes. From soups to marinades and a variety of crockpot recipes, we never thought of broth as containing gluten but it absolutely can. Premade broth, in boxes, tends to be gluten-free and states it clearly on packaging. Bouillon cubes or pastes can have gluten in the ingredient list. If it does not clearly say "gluten-free," read the ingredient list for keywords, or easily order your preferred broth online. We often use the RC Fine Foods Reserve GF paste.

🔎 Where to Find: Broth aisle and Gluten-free food aisle

Soups:

Switch to gluten-free soups (including cream soups) and continue using your current soup and casserole recipes.

Soups have surprised us the most with their inclusion of unexpected gluten. Initially, we eliminated some recipes from our diet because they contained soup (usually a cream soup) for which we could find no gluten-free substitute. Even tomato soup was challenging to find. Recently, however, our local grocery stores have begun carrying specialty brands that offer gluten-free soup options, including cream soups. Many boxed tomato soups are gluten-free. Check your grocery store or online. Pacific Brand, Healthy Valley, Gluten-Free Café, Frontier Soup, and some Progresso soups have options.

🔎 Where to Find: Soup aisle and Gluten-free food aisle

Spices, Oils, and Butter:

> *Most (if not all) spices, oils, and butter are already gluten-free.*

Individual spices (salt, pepper, garlic, oregano, etc) are naturally gluten-free. As previously mentioned, read through combination spice ingredient lists to ensure they are safe. Manufacturers will list ingredients on the label and will identify gluten (wheat, barley, rye, malt) if the spice contains it or may be contaminated.

Oils (olive, vegetable, canola, etc.), butter, and margarine are gluten-free. Just be mindful to prevent cross-contamination (see Chapter 4). Aerosolized spray oils are generally gluten-free unless they're baking sprays that contain flour.

🔎   Where to Find: Spices and Oil aisle

Condiments and Salad Dressing

As covered in Chapter 4, most condiments are gluten-free, and as such, you will experience minimal change with these products. You will likely be able to continue using your same condiments, just prevent cross-contamination and consider using squeeze bottles. Double-check the labels.

🔎   Where to Find: Condiment aisle, International aisle, and Gluten-free aisle

Marinades, Sauces, and Soy Sauce:

> *Gluten-free marinades, sauces, and soy sauce are readily available. Sample different brands for your options.*

For these products, start by reviewing the labels of your favorite brands first and change manufacturers if needed. If you can't find your specific type of sauce/marinade in gluten-free, look online for other versions. We use gluten-free soy sauce in a lot of marinades. For example, San-J Tamari (Japanese soy sauce), Kikkoman gluten-free soy sauce, and La Choy soy sauce have gluten-free options (read the label, stay updated).

🔎 Where to Find: Condiment aisle, International aisle, and Gluten-free aisle

Pasta:

> *Switch to gluten-free pasta and continue with your favorite Italian recipes. Gluten-free pasta will always be clearly labeled.*

The transition from regular pasta to gluten-free pasta has been relatively smooth because of wide availability. The grocery store stocks gluten-free pastas (labeled clearly) in both the regular pasta aisle as well as in the organic/gluten-free section. There are a wide variety of gluten-free pasta styles from spaghetti and fettuccini to macaroni and lasagna.

Similar to flour, gluten-free pasta is created using various flour combinations. For example, one manufacturer's gluten-free fettuccine is made from corn and rice. Another makes linguine from brown rice, amaranth, and quinoa. Other pastas are created from chickpeas or from green lentils and kale. The varieties are endless!

The various flour mixtures result in each pasta's unique taste, texture, and cooking requirements. The primary concern is preventing the pasta from disintegrating, which happens with overcooking. Closely follow the package instructions for best results. The internet is also full of helpful websites and blogs on Italian food and cooking tips for gluten-free pasta. Do yourself a favor and sample a variety of pastas and flours to decide what you like best. We prefer the texture and taste of corn-based pasta.

If you purchase pasta sauce, double-check the ingredient list to ensure there is no gluten. Manufacturers of spaghetti sauce are getting much better at leaving out unnecessary wheat/gluten.

🔍   Where to Find: Pasta aisle and Gluten-free food aisle

> *While researching a future trip, I read an article that said Italy, a country that places such importance on food and socializing, has taken the inclusion of gluten-free options seriously. Italy routinely screens children for celiac disease and provides a state subsidy for the higher cost of gluten-free living. Additionally, Italian law requires schools, hospitals, and public places to offer gluten-free food as a standard. Visit the blog "The Essential Gluten-Free Guide to Italy" by Legal Nomads (https://www.legalnomads.com/gluten-free/italy/) for information and inspiration.*

GLUTEN-FREE SUBSTITUTES – BRANDS TO TRY, GROCERY STORES

_____

_____

_____

_____

_____

_____

_____

_____

_____

_____

_____

_____

_____

_____

_____

_____

GLUTEN-FREE SUBSTITUTES – BRANDS TO TRY, GROCERY STORES

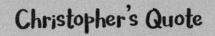

Christopher's Quote

Some fast food restaurants do not offer many gluten-free options. When going out with friends, be prepared by researching restaurants in advance and suggesting two or three popular choices. When in doubt about the safety of my food options, I usually choose a salad and specify no croutons. Or sometimes I just have a soda.

CHAPTER 7 _____

Everyday Gluten-Free Meal and Snack Ideas

As we've said before, changing to a gluten-free diet does not mean you have to create entirely brand-new meals. There are many everyday food options you can still enjoy. Just change one or two things and continue to eat what you love.

Breakfast:

You have many homemade and ready-to-eat choices for breakfast.

- ☞ Cereal: more and more options are becoming available. The following are a few examples (and continue to read labels for latest ingredients):
  - ✓ General Mills: most Chex cereals, most Cheerios cereals, Lucky Charms
  - ✓ Post Cereals: Pebbles cereal including Fruity Pebbles and Cocoa Pebbles (you can use this cereal to make your own version of krispie treats)
  - ✓ Nestlé GoFree brand Corn Flakes, Rice Pops, Coco Rice, and Honey Flakes
  - ✓ Envirokids, Vans, and Erewhon Organic
  - ✓ Examples of cereal that are <u>not</u> currently gluten-free include many brands of cornflake and Rice Krispie-type cereals because they contain malt.

- ☞ Yogurts and cottage cheese. Watch add-in flavoring.
- ☞ Eggs, omelets, and frittatas. Add cheese, vegetables, and meats for added flavor and protein.

☞ Bacon, sausage, and ham. Turkey bacon and meat imitations can sometimes have gluten.

☞ Hash browns (or your own freshly shredded potatoes). If highly processed/seasoned, check the ingredient list.

☞ Gluten-free pancakes and waffles (boxed mix or frozen) are available. Or you can make your own batter using online recipes. Try a variety of brands to see what you like best. Many pancake syrups are gluten-free—like pure maple syrup—but watch out for any syrups containing malt.

☞ French toast (homemade) is a delicious option. For years we avoided this treat because we didn't like the gluten-free bread. However, with thicker bread options now available, we have reintroduced this favorite to our menu. There are several online French toast recipes, including overnight French toast. Tip: We let the gluten-free bread sit out for a few hours to get stale so it soaks up the egg mixture.

☞ Muffins and breakfast breads—either boxed or in the frozen section—are readily available and delicious. Betty Crocker, Krusteaz, and King Arthur offer gluten-free mixes that we enjoy. We like King Arthur Gluten-Free muffin mix for its consistency and because you can add in any extras to the mix—blueberries, chocolate chips, nuts, etc. Adapt your family recipes or look online for new ideas.

☞ Reminder: oatmeal is gluten-free but often processed in facilities that handle wheat and so is often cross-contaminated. Look for a gluten-free label.

☞ Quick Breakfasts: there are several gluten-free options:
   ✓ Ready-to-drink options include Carnation Breakfast Essentials and Ensure shakes. The label should say gluten-free.
   ✓ The ever-increasing protein and granola bar section includes Kind bars, BOBO's Oat Bites, and Nature Valley Protein chewy bars. Be sure any oat-related product says gluten-free.

✓ Frozen breakfast sandwiches/frittatas are available from brands like Udi's and Garden Lites Veggies Made Great (check label). Or you can make your own sandwiches using online recipes.

Lunch and Dinner:

The following is a small sampling of the numerous gluten-free lunch and dinners you can make.

Sandwich Tips:
☞ Choose your favorite gluten-free bread. Many more soft and flexible versions are becoming available.
☞ Use condiments to add moisture and flavor (gluten-free bread is often dry).
☞ Toast the bread for better taste and flexibility.
☞ Most deli meats and cheeses are gluten-free. Check the packaging and talk to the deli manager.
☞ You have endless filling options: deli meats, vegetables, pimento cheese, egg salad, chicken salad, tuna salad, grilled cheese, peanut butter and jelly, etc.

Hot dogs are often gluten-free, and you will find the buns in the frozen bread section. Consider warming the thawed buns in the microwave or buttering them and slowly toasting them in a frying pan or toaster oven for better flexibility and taste.

Hamburger meat is gluten-free, and you can easily add any spices or sauces after double-checking the ingredient list. Warm or toast the hamburger buns for better flavor.

☞ If you're having a cookout, take care to prevent cross-contamination. Keep regular hamburger buns and gluten-free buns physically separated and clearly marked.
☞ Offer condiments from a squeeze bottle instead of a jar.

Chicken options are plentiful.

☞ Grilled, fried, baked, or barbecued. Use gluten-free marinades.

☞ Chicken casserole dishes like chicken and rice, chicken tetrazzini, and chicken parmesan, etc. are all tasty options. Gluten-free panko/breading is readily available as well as gluten-free cream soups often used in recipes.

☞ NOTE: Rotisserie chicken is often contaminated with gluten. Look for a gluten-free label and talk with your deli.

Beef and steak options are endless.

☞ Grill, stir fry, or broil the meat.

☞ Gluten-free natural spices and oils tenderize and add flavor.

☞ If making a pot roast or beef stew with broth and/or packaged seasoning, double-check the label.

☞ Use gluten-free sauces and marinades.

Pork options are still on the table.

☞ Ham, ribs, pork chops, and tenderloins are good options.

☞ Pork barbecue is a delicious meal. Double-check spice ingredients.

☞ Use gluten-free panko rub (or check online for latest options) for pork chops.

☞ Many barbecue sauces are already gluten-free or you can make your own.

Seafood choices are abundantly available.

☞ Shrimp, fish, lobsters, clams, scallops, and oysters are easy to find. Steam, bake, fry, or serve in a casserole.

☞ If frying, be sure the bread coating is gluten-free. Spices like Old Bay are gluten-free (always check the current label).

☞ Any seafood item that is additionally processed (marinated, fried, has a coating, or made into a dip) likely has gluten. Read the ingredient list. You can make these items gluten-free by making them at home with gluten-free substitutions.

Soups are best made from scratch.

☞ As mentioned earlier, many canned soups have gluten. Specialty brands offer a line of gluten-free options. Also check boxed soups.

☞ Use gluten-free broths or bouillon.

☞ Note: if you make chicken noodle soup, add the gluten-free noodles at the end of the cooking process. Overcooked noodles fall apart. As an option, use quinoa instead of noodles.

☞ Hearty soups like homemade chili or bean soup can easily be made gluten-free. Double-check spice ingredients.

Italian Meals:

Italian cuisine converts easily to gluten-free.

☞ Most premade packaged Italian meals at the grocery store contain gluten. For example, store-prepared lasagna, ravioli, carbonara, and meatballs are made with regular ingredients and are not safe. Instead, create your own Italian favorites with the many gluten-free pastas and sauces available.

☞ A variety of gluten-free premade Italian meals are available in the gluten-free frozen section. For example, Udi's makes a delicious ravioli with red sauce, chicken parmesan, and lasagna.

☞ Don't forget the garlic bread! There are a variety of dinner rolls available in the frozen section or you can make your own homemade gluten-free bread (look for online recipes).

☞ Pizza . . . okay. We have to be truthful here. Your journey to find great gluten-free pizza could be a long one, but options are improving. We have tried both making our own homemade gluten-free pizza dough as well as purchasing several different frozen pizzas, and they are an acquired taste. We have, however, found several local pizzerias that make good gluten-free pies. You need to be clear with the establishment that your request for a gluten-free pizza is due to an allergy and talk with them about the precautions they take to ensure no cross-contamination. Some pizzerias are better than others. Also, check the nationwide pizza chains for gluten-free options.

Italian – Dining Out:

We have been pleasantly surprised that many Italian restaurants (and some pizzerias) provide gluten-free entrées and sides. Often these restaurants offer several different pasta options and can adjust for you accordingly. Be sure to speak up and ask if they use separate colanders and prevent cross-contamination.

Mexican Meals:

Fortunately, a wide variety of Mexican dishes are naturally gluten-free. Here are some ideas:
- Tacos (hard shell) are most often made out of corn.
- Soft corn tortillas are gluten-free and labeled as such. Use them for quesadillas, burritos, and enchiladas in place of flour tortillas. TIP: Corn tortillas often fall apart easily, so to avoid this you can either warm the tortilla up in microwave or oven (wrap in a damp towel to keep moist) or even better, spread refried beans or melt shredded cheese between two tortillas and then use them as a taco holder or wrap for a burrito. Frying for 10 seconds per side in a pan with some oil is another good option to prevent it from falling apart.
- Corn tortilla chips are usually safe and labeled.
- Meat, beans, and cheeses are gluten-free. Double-check taco seasoning label or make your own blend.
- Salsa and guacamole are naturally gluten-free. Many queso options are also available or you can make your own.
- Mole sauce can contain gluten, but can also be made gluten-free.
- Gazpacho soup is often gluten-free.

Mexican – Dining Out:

Of all the restaurants we have tried, it has been most difficult to find genuinely gluten-free Mexican establishments. Talk with the restaurant owner and cooks to determine what are safe options. The main problem is cross-contamination in prep areas and shared fryers. For example, the corn chips are usually fried in the same oil as flour tortillas. Upscale Mexican restaurants tend to have more options and follow precautions. We have found large chain restaurants and some small local restaurants offer many gluten-free options. But we've been known to bring in our own chips to safely enjoy the salsa and guacamole.

Asian and Thai Cooking:

There are plenty of gluten-free Asian meal options.

- ☞ Fried rice, rice noodles, and stir-fry options are plentiful and delicious. Where you may have a challenge is with premade sauces like teriyaki, sweet and sour, soy sauce, and pad thai which often have gluten. Switch brands, order online, or make your own sauces to solve the problem.
- ☞ If your recipe calls for batter-fried ingredients, simply use the gluten-free all-purpose flour of your choice.
- ☞ As mentioned earlier, there are plenty of gluten-free soy sauce options.
- ☞ Sushi and many rolls (without tempura or fried crunchies) are gluten-free.

Asian and Thai – Dining Out:

We have had good luck with Asian restaurants that offer many gluten-free options. Again, you have to be clear about your allergy and about needing gluten-free soy sauce, gluten-free broths (if ordering soups), and sauces without wheat/gluten. Assume the restaurant is using soy sauce that has gluten. Ask them about preventing cross-contamination as well (for example, with fried rice). We often bring our own soy sauce as a precaution.

Other Ethnic and Regional Food:

As you can see, we only mention a few varieties of ethnic meals that are easily converted to gluten-free. But there are an amazing array of delicious foods and cooking methods from around the world, and we encourage you to use your knowledge of gluten-free substitutions to keep enjoying these meals. For example, if you love Moroccan, Cuban, Peruvian, Indian, French or Greek cuisines, then learn about the ingredients of the recipes you love, figure out the gluten-free substitution, and be on your way to delicious eating!

Snacks:

We have been amazed by the number of snacks that are already gluten-free.

- ☞ Potato chips, cheese puffs, popcorn, and corn tortilla chips are all gluten-free and will say so on the label. Start with your favorite and review from there. Some specialty-flavored chips do have gluten but check for similar items offered by other manufacturers.
- ☞ There are fewer gluten-free options for crackers and cookies, but alternatives are increasingly available. For these items, start looking in the gluten-free/organic section but be aware they could be in other areas of the store. New options are always arriving. Expect gluten-free pita chips, nut-based crackers, and cheese-based crackers. Pepperidge Farm Gluten-Free Goldfish are available but may need to be

special-ordered. Our latest favorite cracker is by Breton, but Glutino and Lance offer good options.

☞ Most nuts and certain brands of beef jerky are gluten-free, but read labels. Some packaged nuts, like trail mix, or open bins of nuts and mixes will have a label saying "processed in a facility that also processes wheat, etc.". Change to manufacturers who offer these snacks in gluten-free form.

☞ As mentioned previously, gluten-free granola bars and protein bars are readily available and will be clearly labeled.

☞ Remember fruits, vegetables, and cheese snacks are naturally gluten-free!

Baked Goods and Desserts:

Baking gluten-free cakes, cookies, brownies, and any sweet treat is fully possible—whether you are using a gluten-free box mix or converting your own family recipe.

☞ In general, start with your own family recipe (or any recipe) and substitute in gluten-free ingredients. Frequently all you need to do is switch to gluten-free all-purpose flour (with xanthan gum) to get great results. If your results aren't ideal, review the manufacturer's website for tips and help. Sometimes baking with gluten-free flours requires different methods like mixing wet ingredients together before adding dry ingredients. It's also advisable to let a batter sit for a while (or refrigerate) before using and allow baked goods to cool longer on the baking sheet. Follow manufacturer instructions.

☞ Boxed mixes and refrigerated cookie dough are becoming more common in grocery stores and online. They are really delicious.

☞ Many premade gluten-free cookies (like Goodie Girl, Tate's, and Glutino brands) are available and taste great. Take a look in the grocery store cookie aisle, the organic/gluten-free section, and online for options.

Beverages:

Most drinks are gluten-free including soda, juice, sports drinks, flavored water, and milk. Malted chocolate milk or malted milk-shakes contain gluten, but other chocolate milk is safe, just read packaging. Distilled alcohol, regulated by the ATF, is generally gluten-free and gluten-free beer options are growing.

Candy:

Gluten-free candy is readily available. For example, Hershey's chocolate bars, Reese's peanut butter cups (not holiday cups), Three Musketeers, Starburst, Skittles, and Snickers are gluten-free (always read the label to ensure status). Do a "Is _____ gluten-free?" search on your phone and read the ingredients for a quick answer on safety. Usually candy that has cookies, wafers, or krispies (with malt) have gluten. Please note that some surprising candies have gluten, such as gummy bears, licorice, and Twizzlers. Look for a manufacturer with a gluten-free option.

FAVORITE RESTAURANTS WITH GLUTEN-FREE OPTIONS

_____

_____

_____

_____

_____

_____

_____

_____

_____

_____

_____

_____

_____

_____

_____

_____

_____

Christopher's Quote

Making our gluten-free egg noodle recipe helped me understand how the gluten-free flour worked and acted, and how to make the recipe work effectively. Consider using one brand of all-purpose flour in a variety of your recipes - baked goods, gravy, noodles, etc. Then try a different brand of gluten-free flour in the same items to see if you notice a difference in taste or quality. Consider experimenting with newer products as you wish.

CHAPTER 8 ───────────

Christopher's Favorite Recipes

The best way I have dealt with celiac disease is by learning how to cook. I learned a lot from my mom, but I also gained good information from watching cooking channels and YouTube instruction videos. Researching ingredients and how recipes come together helps me fix great meals, and I'm more knowledgeable at restaurants about food options that could potentially have gluten. Staying educated makes me more confident and content with the diet. As you begin cooking gluten-free, we encourage you to start with your own recipes and retrofit them to be your gluten-free favorites. Transitioning to this new lifestyle is already a big change, so keeping things that are familiar to you and your family will make the adjustment easier. When you are ready for new ideas, there are many gluten-free cookbooks and online resources. Don't limit yourself to gluten-free choices only – just about every recipe can be adapted. In this chapter I want to share some family recipes that made my transition to gluten-free much easier.

CHRISTOPHER'S LATKES

This dish is naturally gluten-free, but double-check your spices to ensure they are safe. This recipe makes approximately 6-8 latkes.

Ingredients:
3 - 4 whole potatoes, shredded (or 1/2 package shredded country-style hash browns)
1/4 large yellow onion, chopped
1/2 teaspoon onion powder
1 teaspoon garlic powder
1/2 teaspoon paprika
Cayenne pepper to taste (I use 1/4 teaspoon)
2 eggs
Vegetable oil

Directions:
- ☞ Peel and grate the potatoes, if whole, and place in medium bowl. If using shredded frozen potatoes, thaw completely in the microwave.
- ☞ Place shredded potatoes in a paper towel and squeeze to remove as much moisture as possible.
- ☞ Return potatoes to the bowl and add the rest of the ingredients, except the oil. Mix thoroughly.
- ☞ Turn on the stove to medium heat and place a large nonstick pan on top, fully covered with vegetable oil (about 1/4 inch up the pan).
- ☞ Once the oil is heated to a frying state, use a large spoon and add enough potato mixture to form a 3" diameter cake. Use the spoon to flatten the potato cake to about 1/2-inch thick.
- ☞ Cook the potato cake until it forms a crispy golden-brown crust and flip (around 7 minutes on the first side, but times will vary. Less time on the second side.)
- ☞ Remove from the pan when the other side has a golden-brown crust and place on paper towel.

Latkes topped with fried eggs are delicious.

BISCUITS (AND CINNAMON ROLL BISCUITS)

When I changed to gluten-free, one of the things I missed most was Saturday morning breakfasts which included eggs, bacon, hash browns, and biscuits or cinnamon rolls. We always had nice warm biscuits or rolls, and now those were gone. I researched online the various ways to make biscuits and experimented with gluten-free all-purpose flour and other ingredients. Once the biscuits worked, my mom and I tried to figure out how to make cinnamon rolls using the same dough. They both turned out delicious. This recipe makes 12 biscuits/rolls.

Ingredients:
1 egg
1 cup buttermilk (or pour 1 tablespoon of white vinegar into a measuring cup and fill with milk until it reaches 1 cup)
3 tablespoons whole-milk ricotta or cottage cheese
6 tablespoons unsalted butter, cut into ¼ inch cubes
3 - 4 cups gluten-free all-purpose flour
1 tablespoon baking powder
2 tablespoons sugar

Directions:
- ☞ In a large bowl, whisk together egg, buttermilk, and ricotta cheese. Set aside.
- ☞ In a separate bowl, whisk 3 cups flour, baking powder, and sugar until well blended. Set aside the extra 1 cup of flour as it may be needed to work the dough.
- ☞ Add the cubes of butter to the flour mixture and mix thoroughly with your hands. Mixture will be crumbly. As an alternative you can mix the butter and flour in a food processor to a crumbly consistency.
- ☞ Add the flour and butter mixture to the wet ingredients and thoroughly mix to a dough.
- ☞ Start kneading the dough and slowly add in more flour until it forms a non-sticky dough. Let the dough rest for 10 minutes.
- ☞ Preheat oven to 450 degrees.

☞ Roll the dough to about 1/2-inch thick on a floured surface. Use a biscuit cutter to form even-sized biscuits. Place formed dough touching each other on greased baking pan.

☞ Bake in oven for 15-20 minutes. They will turn a golden brown, but won't rise very tall. Serve with butter and jam.

CINNAMON ROLL BISCUITS

Ingredients:
Use the Biscuits recipe ingredients (page 83), PLUS
4 tablespoons melted butter
1/2 cup light brown sugar
1/2 - 1 teaspoon cinnamon

Icing: (or you can use store bought cream cheese icing)
4 ounces cream cheese (room temperature)
4 tablespoons unsalted butter, softened
1 cup powdered sugar
1 teaspoon vanilla extract
Pinch of salt
1/4 cup milk

Directions
- ☞ Follow the ingredients and instructions for the biscuit recipe through the kneading process (page 83).
- ☞ Preheat oven to 450 degrees.
- ☞ Press out the dough into a large rectangle about 1/4-inch thick on floured surface.
- ☞ Brush the melted butter onto the dough surface. (You will not use all of the butter—just cover the surface).
- ☞ Combine the light brown sugar and cinnamon in a small bowl and thoroughly mix. Evenly sprinkle the sugar and cinnamon mixture on the dough surface in a thin layer. You may not use all of mixture.
- ☞ Starting with the long edge, roll the dough tightly to the long edge. Position the roll seam-side down.
- ☞ Using a serrated knife, cut the rolls to a 1-inch thickness and place touching each other on parchment paper in a greased baking pan. Alternatively, you can place each roll into a greased muffin tin.
- ☞ Bake the rolls for 15-20 minutes. They should be golden brown on top.

☞ For icing, blend together softened cream cheese and butter until combined and smooth (can use hand mixer if you wish). Add vanilla and salt and combine. Whisk in powdered sugar. Add milk slowly (a tablespoon at a time) and mix until thoroughly incorporated. You want a thick but pourable consistency. Store bought cream cheese icing also works well. You can warm it in a microwave for 15-20 seconds and drizzle it on. Enjoy!

GINGER SOY MARINATED FLANK OR SKIRT STEAK

This is a favorite recipe that went away because it had soy sauce in it. When I found soy sauces available in gluten-free (our ONE change), we started using this recipe again. Cook on the grill for the best flavor.

**Note: Double this recipe and use the leftover meat for our Beef Stroganoff.

Ingredients:
1 - 1.5 pounds flank steak or skirt steak (London broil is also an option)
1/4 cup gluten-free soy sauce or tamari
3 tablespoons honey
2 tablespoons apple cider vinegar
1 large clove garlic, crushed
1/2 teaspoon garlic powder
3/4 teaspoon ground ginger
1 tablespoon dried minced onion (or 1/4 cup minced raw onion)
1/4 teaspoon black pepper
1/4 cup olive oil

Directions:
- ☞ Thoroughly mix all ingredients in a bowl. Be sure honey is dissolved.
- ☞ Prepare the meat by piercing it with a fork on both sides. Place the meat flat in a glass casserole dish or in a large plastic leak-proof bag and pour the marinade over it.
- ☞ Marinate overnight in refrigerator and occasionally reposition the meat to season evenly. We recommend 6-12 hours to marinate.
- ☞ Grill or broil the steaks to your liking. Thinly slice.

Serve beef with steamed or roasted vegetables and potatoes.

If you have 2 pounds of steak, double the marinade and prepare and cook the same way. If you have at least half a pound of the cooked beef remaining, save the remainder and cut the meat thinly and into bite-sized pieces. Store it in the refrigerator for the next day's meal of Beef Stroganoff (page 90).

GLUTEN-FREE EGG NOODLES

This homemade egg noodle recipe was passed on from my grandparents and my mom used it for many meals including beef stroganoff, chicken and noodles, and even lasagna. I didn't think I would enjoy noodle dishes again but the gluten-free all-purpose flour with xanthan gum (our ONE change) works very well.

Making the noodles takes some time and can be messy, but it is worth it. I can do all of this by hand with a rolling pin or with a pasta roller. Make the noodles any size you want depending on your recipe.

Ingredients:
(You will need 1 egg and 2/3 cup of flour for every serving/person. This recipe is for 3-4 people.)
3 eggs
1 tablespoon water
2 - 3 cups gluten-free all-purpose flour with xanthan gum
1/4 teaspoon salt
1/4 teaspoon xanthan gum

Directions:
- ☞ In a medium-sized bowl, scramble 3 eggs thoroughly. Mix in water, salt, and xanthan gum.
- ☞ Slowly, starting with 1 cup of flour, add the flour to the egg mixture and stir thoroughly with a fork.
- ☞ Continue to add the flour a few tablespoons at a time until you have formed a dough and it is not sticky. Transfer the dough to a floured surface and knead it until it starts to stick to your hands. Add more flour and start kneading again. Repeat the process of adding flour and kneading until the dough reaches a pliable, yet semi-firm stage. If you create a stiff dough, you will have stiff noodles. You probably will not use all the flour.
- ☞ Let the dough sit covered for 10 minutes.
- ☞ After the dough has rested, dust the work surface with flour and use a rolling pin to spread into a crude circle or rectangle.

Constantly check your rolling pin and beneath the rolled dough to make sure it is not sticking. If it is, add an ample but thin layer of flour. Roll to about 1-2 millimeters thick.

☞ Once the dough is rolled out, let it sit and dry for about 10 minutes (but don't dry out completely – always needs to be pliable). Cut the dough into noodles. The length and width are up to you, but we make each noodle about 1/2-inch wide and about 6-8 inches long.

☞ Cooking the noodles:

> ✓ For the Beef Stroganoff recipe (page 90), bring a large pot of water with 1/2 teaspoon of salt to boil. Gently place noodles into boiling water and gently stir. Cook for about 6 minutes then test a noodle. It should taste like noodle and not dough. If needed, cook an additional minute or two and test again.

> ✓ If using the noodles for a soup or our Chicken and Noodle over Potatoes recipe (page 92), we recommend you boil them in the broth for extra flavor. You can boil the noodles separately and place into the soup, or you can cook them in the soup when it is about 10 minutes from being done. Bring the broth to a boil and cook for 6-8 minutes. Taste test for doneness.

> ✓ For lasagna, there is no need to precook the noodles. Roll the dough to 1-2 millimeters thin. Hand cut the noodles to the size you need based on your pan. To the sauce add one quarter cup of water or wine, and prepare layered lasagna dish as normal. Cook covered for 45 minutes then uncovered for 5-10 minutes. Let stand for 10 minutes before serving.

CROSBY FAMILY BEEF STROGANOFF WITH HOMEMADE EGG NOODLES

My mom learned this recipe from her parents and it is a family favorite. She stopped serving it for about three years until we realized we could make our egg noodles gluten-free. Now we enjoy this dish often.

We frequently use our leftover Ginger Soy Marinated Flank Steak (page 87) in our stroganoff because it is so tender and flavorful. If you do not have time to prepare the beef overnight, you can use a ready-made marinade like Dale's Steak Seasoning. Marinate the meat for 3-4 hours and then grill as usual.

Start with the Gluten-Free Egg Noodles because the whole process takes approximately 1-2 hours. While the egg noodles are resting/drying, begin the beef stroganoff process. Note: If you do not want to make the homemade egg noodles you can substitute with egg tagliatelle gluten-free pasta (Jovial and Schar are two brands that make it).

Step 1: Make the Gluten-Free Egg Noodles
☞   Follow the noodle recipe on page 88. When the dough is made and resting, start the beef stroganoff (below).

Step 2: Make beef stroganoff

Ingredients:
1/2 – 1 pound of cooked, marinated flank steak. The meat should be thinly sliced and in bite-sized pieces.
3/4 cup gluten-free all-purpose flour
1/4 teaspoon paprika
1/2 teaspoon garlic powder
1/2 teaspoon onion powder
1/4 teaspoon salt
1/2 teaspoon pepper
2 tablespoons butter
2 tablespoons olive oil
1 clove garlic, minced

Ingredients (continued):
1/2 cup fresh, sliced mushrooms
1 1/2 - 2 cups gluten-free beef broth
1/2 cup sour cream

Directions:

- ☞ In a gallon bag, combine the flour, paprika, garlic powder, onion powder, salt, and pepper. Mix thoroughly.
- ☞ Add the bite-sized slices of cooked marinated beef to the bag and thoroughly mix, making sure each piece is evenly coated.
- ☞ Place the butter and olive oil in a large pan and heat over medium-high. Once the butter is melted, add minced garlic and sauté about one minute (watch the garlic so it doesn't burn).
- ☞ Place the individual slices of flour-coated beef in the pan (shake off excess flour) and cook each side to a gentle crisp or slight brown (about 3-4 minutes per side).
- ☞ Add mushroom slices and sauté to a soft consistency.
- ☞ Slowly add the beef broth, half a cup at a time, and stir to mix with beef and mushrooms. Continue to add the broth until a gravy sauce forms. You should not need to add extra flour to the gravy but you can if needed. Continue to gently simmer the gravy and beef for approximately 30-45 minutes. You may find that you need to add more broth, or just water, to keep the right consistency. Taste the gravy and season accordingly.
- ☞ While the stroganoff is simmering, go back to the noodles. Roll out the dough as described (page 88, 89) and cut into noodles. Let rest/dry for 10 minutes.
- ☞ Start a large pot of water for the noodles. Add 1/2 teaspoon of salt and bring to a boil. Gently add the cut noodles to the water and stir. Cook for 6 minutes and taste test for doneness.
- ☞ While the noodles are cooking, add the sour cream to the stroganoff about 5-10 minutes before serving and stir thoroughly.
- ☞ Drain the noodles in a colander. Do not rinse.
- ☞ Serve the warm noodles with the beef stroganoff on top. Enjoy.

CHICKEN AND NOODLES OVER POTATOES

This is another recipe from my grandparents and is great to have on cold winter days. You may use any chicken you want, from whole chicken to chicken breasts. We choose to use whole chicken because of the richer taste. Our Gluten-Free Egg Noodles are also perfect in this hearty dish.

Ingredients:
1 whole chicken (3-4 pounds)
1/2 tablespoon kosher salt
1/2 teaspoon black pepper
Fresh (not dried) poultry seasoning pack – sprigs of thyme, rosemary, and sage
1 box gluten-free chicken broth
1 cup sliced carrots
1/2 cup sliced celery
1 small onion, quartered
2 cloves garlic, crushed
2 bay leaves
2 teaspoons garlic powder
1/2 teaspoon oregano
Salt and pepper to taste

Additions to this meal:
- ✓ Make Gluten-Free Egg Noodles (page 88) but cook them in this broth for extra flavor.
- ✓ Make or buy prepared mashed potatoes.

Directions:
- ☞ Rinse and pat dry the whole chicken. Be sure to take out any gizzards. If there is excess fat/skin around neck area, cut it out and discard.
- ☞ Place whole chicken in a large pot for boiling. Add the carrots, celery, onion, garlic, and bay leaves. Pour in box of chicken broth, then add enough water to cover chicken. Add the salt, pepper, thyme, rosemary, and sage.

☞ Bring the water with the chicken to a boil with medium-high heat then cover and simmer on low-medium for 1 1/2 - 2 hours. The internal temperature should be 165 degrees.

☞ Begin making the Gluten-Free Egg Noodle recipe. Have noodles cut and ready.

☞ Begin making mashed potatoes per your own recipe or use ready-made mashed potatoes (that are gluten-free).

☞ Once chicken is fully cooked, carefully remove it and let cool slightly. Take off the skin and shred the chicken meat and set aside.

☞ Taste test the remaining broth (when cooled a little). If desired, add salt and pepper as well as garlic powder and oregano. Discard the bay leaves, sprigs of thyme, rosemary, and sage. If you wish you can skim off some of the excess fat on top with a spoon.

☞ Bring the broth to a boil over medium-high heat. Add the noodles to the broth and cook for 6-7 minutes. Taste test for doneness.

☞ Reduce heat to low/medium. Add the shredded chicken to the broth with noodles and reheat for a few minutes.

☞ To serve, use a shallow bowl and place mashed potatoes on bottom. Spoon broth with vegetables, chicken, and noodles on top of potatoes. Enjoy.

WELCOME TO THE NEIGHBORHOOD CAKE

My family loves this chocolate cake. My mom says she got the recipe from a neighbor who made it for us when we moved into a new house. After we found gluten-free chocolate cake mix (our ONE change), we gave it a try. Success!

Ingredients:
1 box gluten-free chocolate cake mix
1 small box chocolate pudding mix (read label - most are gluten-free)
1 3/4 cup milk
2 large eggs
3/4 cups mini chocolate chips (read label – most are gluten-free)

Directions:
- ☞ Preheat the oven to 350 degrees.
- ☞ In a large bowl, combine the cake mix, milk, and eggs. Use a hand mixer to thoroughly mix ingredients, about 2-3 minutes.
- ☞ Add the chocolate pudding mix and use the hand mixer again about 1 minute. Batter will be thick.
- ☞ Add the mini chocolate chips to the batter and blend in using a large spoon.
- ☞ Spray a Bundt pan with oil.
- ☞ Pour the batter evenly into the Bundt pan and place the pan into the heated oven.
- ☞ Bake the cake for approximately 50 - 60 minutes. Test the cake after 50 minutes with a knife. You want it to pull out fairly clean with only some chocolate chip residue.
- ☞ Let the cake cool. Loosen the sides and center with a knife and when cooled, flip onto a large plate.
- ☞ This cake does not need icing, but you can drizzle chocolate sauce or sift powdered sugar on top.

TAILGATE PUMPKIN CAKE

Every fall when we would tailgate at football games, my mom would make this really great pumpkin cake. The gluten-free all-purpose flour (our ONE change) allowed us to keep this dessert. It tastes exactly like the regular recipe and does not fall apart. Here's the recipe:

Ingredients:
4 large eggs
1 cup canola oil
15-ounce can of pumpkin
1 1/3 cup sugar
2 cups gluten-free all-purpose flour with xanthan gum
1 teaspoon xanthan gum (if your flour does not include it)
1 teaspoon baking soda
2 teaspoons baking powder
1 teaspoon salt
1/2 teaspoon ground ginger
2 teaspoons cinnamon
Cream cheese frosting (gluten-free)

Directions:
- ☞ Preheat oven to 350 degrees.
- ☞ In a large bowl, beat together eggs and oil with an electric mixer.
- ☞ Add the pumpkin and sugar to the egg mixture and blend thoroughly.
- ☞ In a separate bowl, thoroughly combine flour, baking powder, baking soda, salt, ginger, and cinnamon.
- ☞ Slowly add the flour mixture to the wet mix and blend with a mixer. Note sometimes the batter gets weirdly thick due to the xanthan gum. It's okay and just the nature of baking gluten-free. You can mix by hand if you wish.
- ☞ Grease a 9" x 13" glass or metal pan. Pour the pumpkin batter into the pan and spread evenly.
- ☞ Bake the cake for 30 minutes. Test doneness with a knife or toothpick.
- ☞ Cool the cake. Spread on cream cheese frosting, if desired.

YOUR FAMILY RECIPES – GLUTEN-FREE

_____

_____

_____

_____

_____

_____

_____

_____

_____

_____

_____

_____

_____

_____

_____

_____

_____

YOUR FAMILY RECIPES – GLUTEN-FREE

_____

_____

_____

_____

_____

_____

_____

_____

_____

_____

_____

_____

_____

_____

_____

_____

_____

_____

_____

_____

YOUR FAMILY RECIPES – GLUTEN-FREE

_____

_____

_____

_____

_____

_____

_____

_____

_____

_____

_____

_____

_____

_____

_____

_____

_____

_____

_____

_____

HELPFUL RESOURCES ──────────

The following is a listing of some online resources that can help you with your transition to a gluten-free diet and update you on the latest research. *Please note we are not endorsing the websites and we are not endorsed by these organizations.* We encourage you to use internet resources with caution, and always talk directly with your physician and dietician for assistance with your diet and medical care.

Beyond Celiac *www.beyondceliac.org*
Celiac Disease Foundation *www.celiac.org*
Food Allergy Research & Education *www.foodallergy.org*
Gluten Intolerance Group   *www.gluten.org*
National Celiac Association   *www.nationalceliac.org*

In addition to websites, also check social media portals for local and national resources that are available to you. Simply type in "celiac disease" or "gluten-free" in the search bar and you will find a variety of support groups, blogs, and other helpful resources.

Finally, please join our community by following us on social media. You will find us on Instagram (@celiaclost) and Facebook as "Celiac Lost". Visit our website at www.celiaclost.com. We would love to hear from you and share our tips, tricks, and inspiration while on this gluten-free journey!

ACKNOWLEDGMENTS ———————

We have many people we want like to thank for their help and support of this book.

First we want to thank my dear friends Elisabeth Sandberg, Marion Eledge, Alicia Vance and Kim Coggin for being our beta readers. Your time and honest feedback were invaluable and helped set us in the right direction.

Thank you to my husband, Greg Shiflett, for his time, support, and critique, and for providing the invaluable resources to get this project done. Thank you, Tyler Shiflett, for reviewing and approving. We hope we will make you proud!

Thank you to my sister, Suzan Fischer, for reviewing and providing feedback on the book. I always appreciate your love and support.

Thank you to my friend, Vicki Vogt, for additional editorial help and improvement.

Thank you to our friend, Mandie Nimitz, who provided us with important insight and reflection, and helped us focus our vision for the book and related social media. Your help has resulted in a much better project.

BIBLIOGRAPHY

Celiac Disease. (2014, October). *Pediatrics in Review*,
    35(10), 409-416.[1]
Data you need to eat smartly (n.d.). In *Gluten
    Free Watchdog.org*. Retrieved from https://
    www.glutenfreewatchdog.org/about[2]
Frequently asked questions about food allergies. (2017,
    December 18). In *FDA*. Retrieved from https://
    www.fda.gov/Food/IngredientsPackagingLabeling/
    FoodAllergens/ucm530854.htm
Labeling policies. (2019, July 8). In *United States
    Department of Agriculture*. Retrieved from https://
    www.fsis.usda.gov/wps/portal/fsis/topics/
    regulatory-compliance/labeling/Labeling-Policies
Living with Celiac Disease (n.d.). In *beyondceliac.org*.
    Retrieved from https://www.beyondce-
    liac.org/living-with-celiac-disease/
Major food allergen labeling for wines, distilled spirits, and malt
    beverages (2012, September 4). In *TTB.gov*. Retrieved from
    https://www.ttb.gov/labeling/major-food-allergen-labeling
The essential gluten-free guide to Italy (2019, June). Retrieved
    from https://www.legalnomads.com/gluten-free/italy/
What is celiac disease? (n.d.). In celiac.org. Retrieved from https://
    celiac.org/about-celiac-disease/what-is-celiac-disease/

---

1   Used in the explaining the list of gluten-free food
2   This private website tests products to determine if their gluten-free claims are
    accurate and if the manufacturer adheres to gluten-free safety standards. A
    monthly subscription is required to see test results.

Made in the USA
Monee, IL
02 July 2020